Self Care Guide

For Beginners

Learn How toCreate Your Own Self-Care Plan to Nourish Your Mind, Body and Spirit, So You Can Show Up As Your Best Self

By Joan Dermody

Contents

Thank you for buying this book and I hope that you will find it useful. If you will want to share your thoughts on this book, you can do so by leaving a review on the Amazon page, it helps me out a lot.

Introduction

Life would be so much simpler if you loved yourself. A lot of individuals deal with low self-esteem. A lot of other individuals are merely uncaring towards themselves. When was the final time your mom asked if you were 'taking care of yourself'? Can you truthfully claim that you are?

Frequently, we put excessive pressure on ourselves. We are continuously striving towards our objectives, and we beat ourselves up in case we are anything less than ideal during that pursuit. Is it any shock we are frequently over-tired, depressed and malnourished?

What a distinction it would make if you took care of yourself. In case you surrounded yourself with buddies who liked you, if you provided yourself a break every once in a while, and if you informed yourself that you were doing terrific.

What if you actually liked who you were, and you were pleased with what you have? Easy: you'd be satisfied. You'd be healthier, more pleased, and more satisfied. And that sensation would radiate from you and impact everybody you communicated with.

In this guide, we are going to see that this needs a two-pronged attack. We have to alter our thinking and how we think about ourselves, and we likewise have to alter the manner in which we care for ourselves. What we consume, how we invest our time, and how we manage our environment.

I compare this to caring for yourself how a mom may care for her kids. That indicates not just looking after yourself physically by grooming, feeding, and ensuring that whatever else is done right—however, likewise, looking after yourself mentally. When you're down, a great mom is going to inform you not to fret, that you're excellent. In case we treated ourselves such as this and internalized that type of love, the world would be a less complicated, kinder location.

Every chapter in this book is going to deal with one of these elements, and by the conclusion, we are going have a plan of self-care that is going to nurture our wellbeing and soul!

Chapter 1: CBT and Mindfulness

Initially, we begin by altering the manner in which we speak to ourselves. And this starts with CBT and mindfulness.

CBT, or Cognitive Behavioural Therapy, is the preferred method in clinical psychology and it will be among the most vital tools within this guide for changing the manner in which we see ourselves.

Today all counselors are utilizing CBT. While it's most likely just a matter of time prior to a brand-new school appearing and knocking CBT off the leading place, it still represents an effective tool that the NHS and numerous others have actually utilized to inexpensively and rapidly enhance the lives of countless clients. The 'rapidly and inexpensively' parts are likewise important as they indicate that anybody can use the concepts and see instant benefit, enhancing their self-confidence without any requirement to shell out a ton of cash and time on therapy.

Clearly, if your signs continue, you ought to look for expert assistance, however, up until then, you can attempt some Do It Yourself to see if CBT is what you require to enhance your self-concept.

A Short History

Basically, CBT is made up of 2 ideas-- cognitive psychology and behaviorism. Behaviourism is a traditional idea that claims how we find out how to associate an occasion with a result to such a level that we can start dealing with the occasion as a result.

For instance, in Pavlov's popular experiment utilizing dogs, he instructed his dog subjects to drool at the noise of the bell by getting them accustomed to listening to the bell as they consumed food.

This relates to your self-confidence, because you can wind up having physical responses to conditions in which you're placed under pressure. For instance, you may discover that in social scenarios, you find yourself perspiring or sweating, as through your experience, you have actually started to associate them with causing humiliation or embarrassment. Additionally, you may find yourself feeling sluggish or depressed when you're trying something brand-new if you have actually fallen short numerous times in the past. Here the bad results serve as 'reinforcement', telling you that your aspirations are destined to fail. This is a learning system that typically assists us to stay clear of making errors and which is typically adaptive in many scenarios. In contemporary society, nevertheless, there are times when it could be mentally destructive.

Behavioral treatment to treat such associations includes 'reassociation.' This would suggest training yourself to find out that placing yourself out on a limb can result in favorable results as well. You may accomplish this by going to great deals of social settings that you understand you'll take pleasure in, or by attempting great deal of brand-new things that you believe you'll be proficient at.

You ought to likewise make certain you surround yourself with beneficial individuals who are going to compliment and motivate you instead of dragging you down. By doing this, you are going to likewise be getting consistent support that you're a capable and valuable individual.

Because of behaviorism, however, psychology has actually carried on understanding that there is a conscious element in a lot of our issues. This is the vital contribution that CBT makes by presenting a cognitive element to our mind and our nervousness.

When it comes to issues such as low self-confidence, the cognitive element might be unfavorable ruminations in which you consider how every little thing is going to misfire, talking yourself out of doing things or unfavorable self-talk.

Chapter 2: Dealing With the Inner Critic

Clients with low self-confidence are going to typically explain how they have a 'little voice' in the rear of their head continuously informing them they will fall short. Other principles in CBT are 'overgeneralization', where you presume that due to the fact that you have actually fallen short at one thing, you will fall short at all activities, and 'false hypotheses', where you improperly anticipate that you will fall short at your duties. We are going to be utilizing CBT strategies so as to assist to conquer this insecurity.

Mindfulness

CBT professionals have actually designed numerous approaches that you can utilize to fight these issues. Among the most typically utilized of these is really obtained from meditation and is called 'mindfulness.' Clients are advised to discover a peaceful location and to take a seat with their eyes closed. Similar to meditation, they are then advised to assess their internal thoughts.

This does not suggest that they ought to try to clear their minds; nevertheless, rather they are advised to simply 'monitor' ideas as they go by without participating in them, simply noticing the content of their brains as they may view clouds passing in the sky. In this manner, they may determine the sort of things they are assuming and particularly any damaging ideas they may be having.

As clients improve at this, they are expected to be in a position to do it throughout daily activities, and after that, step in; finding the destructive and unfavorable ideas and seeing them for what they are.

A lot of unfavorable ruminations are senseless, and even if they aren't, they definitely do more damage than good, so finding out how to find them, and after that, put an end to them is an important ability. Likewise, to assist in this culture of mindfulness, clients are invited to keep journals of their activities and thoughts -- then to go through them and observe how anything they have actually done or said might be bothersome to their self-image.

Good Self-Talk

You can additionally counter these unfavorable thoughts with favorable ones, making use of 'positive self-talk' to declare your worth. Here you ought to ensure to concentrate on your good points, and to keep in mind compliments you might have gotten previously. Rather than informing yourself you're fat continuously, substitute this with pointers about your straight teeth or great eyes. You'd be amazed by how helpful this could be.

Hypothesis Checking

Patients are additionally informed to engage in 'hypothesis testing', where they are urged to evaluate their incorrect hypotheses, ideally understanding that they are unproven. For instance, if a client is terrified to talk in public since they are worried they'll stutter and fall short, then they are urged to, in fact, attempt speaking in public to discover if this is the case. Generally, they'll discover it isn't. This additionally works to protect against overgeneralization, and once again, as a method to counter any unfavorable associations they have actually established.

So, if you're struggling with low self-confidence, then you may wish to attempt utilizing these guidelines. Ensure you keep on heading out and challenging yourself, even if you truly are less than competent at what it is you wish to attain, this is the only method with which you will get better.

Ending up being reclusive is going to just offer you more time to ponder and send you into a descending spiral. Likewise, surround yourself with favorable buddies and associates and attempt to concentrate on the excellent elements of what you do. Support yourself with good self-talk and attempt to capture yourself having unfavorable thoughts and mark them out. In case this still does not work, then it's maybe time to look for aid from an expert who may talk you through the procedure.

Chapter 3: Self-Fulfilling Prophecies

A self-fulfilling prophecy explains an occurrence whereby what you think to be real can really come true by the reality that you, in fact, believe it or that other individuals believe it. If this sounds complex, then picture an instance. Suppose you're a kid at school who has an older sibling who just recently had an identical teacher and proved really effective.

By this reality alone, the other students and teachers are going to presume that this brand-new kid is going to get excellent grades too. This expectation and self-confidence will, in-turn, rub off on him, and he'll begin to see himself as somebody who has the terrific academic capability. (This is likewise an ideal instance of how influences beyond our control can form who we are-- and the reason why it is so crucial to take things back into our own hands!).

As you're most likely informed, you have a tendency to like things that you do good in; therefore, by believing you're proficient at academia you are going to then begin to delight in it more, and place in more time because of this. This is why sports psychologists utilize the 'sandwich' method when offering criticism.

By doing this, they may get their recommendations across without harming the esteem of the gymnast or sprinter. For that reason, you have to attempt and continuously boost your own self-confidence and carefully control how you view yourself so as to boost your success.

The Law of Attraction

How you view yourself likewise speaks volumes to other individuals as you are going to expose your confidence in subtle manners-- the manner in which you walk, the manner in which you talk and the manner in which you dress and the manner in which you behave. If you act as though you are worthy of respect, then you'll begin to think it yourself and if you begin to believe it, then so are going to others.

This, in fact, goes much deeper than abstract viewpoints, nevertheless and can even be utilized to produce success and wealth. For instance, by dressing effectively and putting on great watches (knock-offs are going to do, nobody is going to know), you become able to pay for them. If you project a picture of being rich, then others are going to start to believe you're effective and rich. This can imply that your boss is more probable to offer you a promotion. It likewise implies others are going to be more probable to trust you in business and that other rich people are going to gravitate towards you. Even the presents you get are going to be more costly usually as you usually have a tendency to spend more on presents for individuals who own more costly things-- otherwise, it will not fit with the design and you'll look inexpensive. If you act positively with the other sex, then they are going to presume you remain in high need, and as such, are going to discover you more appealing.

So dressing properly can make other folks think you are effective and that may make you feel effective as well. Do not simply look the part, however, act the part, and in time, by imitating the behavior and actions of somebody effective, you'll begin to pick them up as routines.

Chapter 4: Taking Care Of Your Appearance

Among the most significant reasons why lots of people experience low self-confidence is that they're dissatisfied with a physical feature. In case this is you, then you ought to be delighted to understand that there is a great deal you may do, and there's a sporting chance you're not optimizing your capacity. Here's how to start resembling a million dollars.

It's the Small Things

To start, looks are not always about your face, and for lots of guys, particularly low self-confidence can come from not being as tall as they want to be. Even if this isn't a specific source of contention for you, including a bit of additional height is going to instantly assist you to feel more positive as you look down on individuals, instead of continuously looking up.

However, it's difficult to make yourself grow taller, right? Yes and no. Essentially, instead of really growing taller yourself, you may make yourself seem taller by purchasing insoles that boost your height. In case you type into e-bay 'high insoles', you'll discover numerous items along the lines of what you're searching for. These only cost a little and could be quickly slipped within your shoe, and then adapted to be shorter or taller as much as approximately 4 inches.

4 inches of additional height in case the shoes you're using enable it, take you from 5'9 to a relatively high 6'1. In case you mix this with relatively big shoes, you could actually be rather high. For ladies, the identical could be correct of high heels, and as an included perk, these likewise make ladies look taller and enhance their stride and gait.

For guys bulking up is going to likewise make you more enforcing, and as you usually fill up more area, you'll feel more positive and commanding. Attempt consuming big quantities of protein together with routine physical exercise and work specifically on your shoulders and chest to develop an enforcing shape.

It's difficult to feel unconfident when you're more than 6 feet and covered in muscle. At the identical time, guys who are mindful about their weight ought to ensure to do a great deal of aerobic exercise and stay clear of fatty meals to get themselves feeling less chubby and leaner.

Similarly, for ladies, toning your abs and firming up your backside can make you feel sexier, and once again, enhance your shape. To assist you in the process, you can constantly utilize underclothing that keeps in the fatter parts and plumps out the bits that require plumping. Corsets and girdles are the most ideal, however, you can likewise get trousers that sustain your bottom. Girdles likewise exist for men and while it might be a tad humiliating, they can, at the identical time, make you feel more self-assured when you're out.

Posture

You understand what likewise makes a big distinction to the manner in which you feel? Posture.

In the previous part, we saw the strength of feeling bigger or taller. This may make you physically use up more room, which consequently can significantly increase self-confidence. However, just by pulling your shoulders back and holding your chin up, you can have a really comparable impact. Not just that, however, this has a physiological effect on your state of mind, which assists you to feel more encouraging.

Having Your Best Face On

Placing extra lifts within your shoes may all be a bit severe, however, if it's simply your facial functions you're worried about, there's still a lot you can do without turning to surgical treatment. To start, ensure you obtain a haircut and one which matches the shape of your head.

The squarer your jaw, the more rounded a cut you are going to require and vice versa as a basic guideline. In case you're male, you likewise have to think of facial hair, and while this is usually a style error, it can often actually enhance your appearance -- simply take a look at Rowan Atkinson in Mr. Bean compared to the identical person in Blackadder. You may likewise wish to attempt dying your hair to observe if another color matches you more effectively.

If you're a lady, you have the advantage of having the ability to boost your features with cosmetics. This indicates utilizing foundation to cover blemishes and spots and blusher to deliver a tad more color to the cheeks. Typically those who are a bit shy are going to attempt to use makeup minimally so as not to accentuate themselves. Nevertheless, this effort to 'conceal' in plain sight can trigger all the identical self-fulfilling prophecy effects that we have actually formerly looked into. To put it simply, you shrink away, and individuals presume that you do not wish to be seen.

If you get expert suggestions on how to do your makeup, you may optimize your excellent features and up your allure, even in case you can't assist your natural charm. An expert from someplace such as 'Color Me Beautiful' is going to inform you not just which colors match you finest, however, likewise what your finest features are.

Usually, you are going to be informed to concentrate on either your lips or eyes, depending upon which is your more powerful feature, and after that, to administer the heaviest quantity of cosmetics here to draw the eyes to your properties and far from your imperfections.

So in case you have great lips, you may be recommended to utilize a bit of bright red lipstick to make them appear more welcoming and fuller, while in case you're greatest feature is your eyes, you may be advised to utilize eye liner or eye shadow to make them stand apart. Typically, it's ideal not to go to large on both as you can wind up appearing like an adult movie star or as if you're simply attempting too hard, and while your colors ought to be strong, they should not look as if you're using face paint-- natural-looking colors that match your complexion are recommended.

Want a more natural appearance? That's great too-- however, that does not indicate not utilizing any cosmetics whatsoever. It simply suggests being more subtle, and thoroughly emphasizing your finest features.

Grooming

Both females and males ought to likewise ensure they groom effectively. For ladies, that indicates eliminating any stray facial hairs and moisturizing routinely. For guys, that once again suggests moisturizing to eliminate dead skin along with trimming their ear hairs and nasal hairs, which could be really nasty in case it is overlooked. Simultaneously, utilize whitening toothpaste, and perhaps even a particular whitener to provide your teeth a radiance.

Additionally, a better set of glasses or a cool set of sunglasses can enhance your face and make you look cool or smart, depending upon your preferred appearance. Invest a bit more in the important things that you utilize to adorn and decorate your face.

Essentially, the take-home message is not to quit on your appearance. So long as you place effort into your look and ask buddies for truthful guidance, you'll look nicer and feel greater about yourself. There's absolutely nothing bad with cutting a couple of corners or utilizing a couple of tricky techniques to enhance the manner you look, and in case you look great, you'll feel great.

It's not even practically the manner in which you appear because of your grooming-- it's likewise about the manner in which it makes you feel. Making an effort to take care of yourself is a physical pointer that you do appreciate your appearance. This is an opportunity to relax, and the sensation of running a razor across your skin and opening those pores could be very cathartic-- like you're releasing the day's tensions.

Why not invest a bit more in a sophisticated bathroom and buy a walk-in shower, and even a jacuzzi? You might obtain a steam bath and turn your house into a tiny spa.

Spa breaks themselves likewise are extremely suggested for both men and women. Having somebody mindful of your requirements, being spoiled, and leaving smelling and appearing excellent, these all make a substantial distinction to the manner in which you feel, look and present yourself!

Chapter 5: Looking After Your Health

One foolproof manner to enhance your self-confidence is by working out. The apparent reason why this works is since you'll enhance your body, which is going to make you more appealing. You will not feel as physically intimidated by other individuals, you'll win regard from others who are impressed by your brand-new shape or jealous even (you'll discover that you end up being a font of understanding for anybody who wishes to do the identical), you'll be greater at sports and all exercises, and you'll be more appealing to the different sex.

That's not all working out has to do with, nevertheless. If you train routinely, you'll quickly discover that it impacts you in the manner in which you would not have actually anticipated. Training your body is a thing you may do frequently that has a useful and noticeable impact. Gradually, you are going to see that you're managing an element of yourself. Each time you go to the gym, you leave a bit better than you were prior, and that's one beneficial thing you have actually performed that day. Additionally, when you remain in the gym, attempting to run an additional mile on the treadmill or raise an additional pound on the bench press, you're proving yourself and becoming greater.

You're challenging yourself and conquering it daily-- with time, you'll find out that you may do the identical in any element of your life. Exercising is really a life-affirming activity that can assist you in growing both physically and psychologically.

Exercising is going to likewise boost your state of mind, therefore your self-confidence, in other ways too. The real act of exercising triggers your body to launch the feel-good hormonal agent serotonin. In addition to that, it likewise results in neurogenesis, the birth of brand-new brain cells. In other words, training is going to raise your state of mind and enhance your cognitive efficiency both instantly and with time.

Getting Going With a Fitness Program

To start training, then you have to examine your present condition. In case you're presently chubby, you have to be doing big quantities of aerobic exercise and cutting your calorie consumption. If you're presently extremely thin, you have to do the reverse-- utilizing fewer reps with a heavier weight while boosting the quantity of protein you consume.

You may even take either a weight gainer or a protein shake to enhance your eating plan. Likewise, to reduce weight, you have to train more frequently-- about 5 times a week, however; to get bigger and stronger, you have to train more intensely and less frequently to provide your muscles time to develop and recuperate.

To start, you can train utilizing an easy full-body regimen. While 'split' regimens and so forth are more helpful to training when you're more advanced, to begin with, you have to get your body accustomed to training.

Each session ought to last approximately forty minutes, and each exercise ought to be done for 3 sets. When you start to see development, start reading and discover the methods and tips utilized by the pros.

The most vital thing, however, is that you discover a program, and after that, stay with it. Even if that program isn't ideal, it is going to bring some outcomes merely because of the truth that you're doing some sort of training. That likewise indicates it's far better to do a thing 2 or 3 times a week, instead of being too eager immediately. Consistency is what truly matters here.

Diet and Sleep

Nutrition can make a big distinction to the manner in which you feel about yourself and your state of mind generally. That's partially since your eating plan is going to have an effect on your appearance and your energy.

Foods which contain vitamin C, for instance, are going to enhance your state of mind due to the fact that they supply an increase of serotonin-- vitamin C being utilized to create serotonin. Also, foods high in tryptophan are going to do the identical thing.

Practically any food is going to set off a release of dopamine, the reward hormone. On the other hand, in case you do not eat frequently, you are going to have high cortisol causing anxiety and stress.

Foods high in magnesium, zinc, and vitamin D (to name a few) can all assist in boosting testosterone creation, which in males and females is carefully related to boosted state of mind, drive, and energy.

Alternatively, however, foods that are high in processed sugars can trigger low-level swelling. This is regulated through the launch of pro-inflammatory cytokines, that can likewise impact the brain. Ever questioned why you feel down when you have a stomach bug or a cold? Brain swelling is potentially the culprit!

Processed foods and simple sugars (specifically acellular carbohydrates) can likewise adversely affect the 'gut microbiome'. This suggests that they can feed the bad germs that reside in our guts and starve the good ones. That, consequently, has a huge influence on energy and mood, viewing as these germs launch various hormones and neurotransmitters, and play a huge part in basal metabolism.

Sweet foods likewise spike the blood with insulin and sugar, which then rapidly dissipates. This leads to a 'crash' where blood sugar level is low and cortisol is high once again. Naturally, processed, simple sugars likewise usually do not include healthy nutrients, which indicates you do not get all the mood and hormone boost you receive from the excellent things.

So in case you wish to feel excellent, then you have to consume well. Treat yourself yes, however, do so by utilizing fruits, yogurts, veggies, and other healthy things. By doing this, you'll feel much better in the short long term.

Sleep is just as crucial. Sleeping inadequately is going to trigger your physical looks to degrade, in addition to your psychological health and your state of mind. Bad sleep triggers bags beneath the eyes, blotchy-red skin, bloodshot eyes, and the wear and tear of nails and hair in time. It likewise results in weight gain.

In the short-term, bad sleep is going to leave you with low energy, and is going to boost tension hormones such as cortisol and adrenaline. You'll be wired, fraught and nervous.

The option is to sleep better and longer! Consider this an essential element of your self-care, that is going to assist you to feel and look your finest.

Here are some essential suggestions to think about:

- Get at least 8 hours each night

- Goal to head to bed at the identical time every night. Our bodies like predictability.

- Discover your own 'chronotype' by exploring. What times work ideally for you to sleep and awaken?

- Take a hot shower or bath prior to bed

- No screens 1 hour prior to bed. Go through a book and attempt to remain calm. This is 'unwinding' time.

We can likewise utilize a bit of CBT to go to sleep much faster. Rather than fretting about not getting adequate sleep or attempting to push yourself to sleep, rather concentrate on simply delighting in the relaxation. The paradox is that when you carry this out, you drop off to sleep much quicker!

Chapter 6: Dealing With Regret

Regretting the past is a thing that all of us understand we should not do-- and that all of us understand is useless-- and yet all of us still likewise tend to do it.

Regrettably, being sorry for mistakes is a thing that is mainly out of our control. We are configured to gain from mistakes due to the fact that in the wild, it would have assisted us to stay clear of making comparable errors in the future. We lament touching fire basically as quickly as we try it, and hence we are really unlikely to the identical thing two times.

However, in our history, our errors tended to be far more well-defined and preventable in the future. The errors we make today have a tendency to be more complex and dwelling on them has a tendency to be less beneficial.

Let's take that man or woman you liked 10 years back, for example. They were providing clear indicators of interest and desired you to flirt, however, you were too shy. You have actually carried on ever since, and you're gladly in a brand-new relationship, however, it does not prevent you from being sorry for that previous error.

Similarly, you may have slipped up in your profession one time. Perhaps you lost an essential file which lost the business thousands, which resulted in you being demoted. Or possibly you slipped up when you shouted at your buddy in haste. These are errors you can't 'reverse' and that you understood were not good during the time-- no future success will eliminate them, and they are going to keep repeatedly playing in your mind up until you go crazy. Or will they?

Does Time Heal Regrets?

If you're reading this chapter, it's most likely due to the fact that you're dealing with some regret, whether it was a little recent error or a huge mess up, then you're most likely hoping that I will inform you it disappears. I wish I could, however sadly, the proof isn't so apparent.

According to one research study by Gilovich et al., released in Psychological Review, some remorses are going to recover in time, however, others are going to be less probable to do so. That's due to the fact that there are 2 kinds of regret: regrets of omission and commission. Remorses of commission are regarding things you did, while remorses of omission are regarding things you did refrain from doing.

Which ones last the longest? That's correct-- we are sorry for the stuff we do not do for longer, and as a matter of fact, those remorses have a tendency never ever to recover. This appears like an obvious message to 'do more things', however, once again, it's most likely a bit more complex than that.

The initial thing I saw when thinking of this study was that opportunities you didn't take have a tendency to be simpler to correct than those you did. 'That which has actually been done, can not be reversed.' To put it simply, if you're lamenting refraining from doing something, then an apparent answer is to merely do it now. Get the phone and start speaking with the one who got away!

The other point to think about is that the entire idea of 'paths not taken' is one that is rather unreasonable at its finest. We regret the things we do not do since we never ever know. We have an idealized variation of how those things would have ended up in our minds, so we are sorry for not living that feasible truth. On the other hand, the important things we did do, we got to see plainly-- hence they have a tendency to be substantially less intriguing.

Let's suppose you constantly wished to transfer to Australia as a kid. You pick not to since you hesitate, you do not have the cash, you believe it's reckless, and so on, and hence you devote the rest of your years questioning what it would have been like and being sorry for your choice not to.

You might have done numerous other amazing things in your life-- whether that's marrying and having kids, being there to support your loved ones, or whatever, the issue is that you understand what that felt like and it was sketchy. Hence the 'undone' things constantly appear more fascinating. Similarly, the errors you make you endure, therefore, you determine they might never ever have actually been that bad.

And what you likewise need to understand, is that it's really vital that you do turn down a portion of what life has to provide. Really frequently so as to experience something, we need to always refuse something else. There are billions of choices available to you each and every single moment, and yet you are going to constantly simply pick one of them.

This may sound dismal-- as if you'll never ever be happy with what you choose-- and it's quite an instance of 'the grass is constantly greener.' However, what I'm actuuually stating is that the lawn constantly appears greener. It's not, and what you have actually done is most likely completely rewarding and amazing in its own right: you simply need to find out how to notice that.

In case you can reframe the manner in which you view your paths 'untaken' then, you may discover that you can conquer that sensation of remorse. However, would they fade gradually as time moved forward even if you never ever managed this, or does the research study demonstrate that they aren't ever going to disappear?

To be sincere, the research study appears to recommend that our remorses will not totally fade-- and especially when they're connected to things we didn't do. However, I heard a good method of taking a look at this just recently when viewing Vsauce video on YouTube. In an episode entitled 'Mistaeks', the speaker paraphrases a buddy of his. That buddy informed him that previous errors resembled carvings in a tree. They do not grow with the tree-- they do not even get greater. Nor do they have a tendency to vanish, and as a matter of fact, in many cases, they can become darker.

Nevertheless, while the marks do not alter, the tree does, and gradually, it grows to end up being considerably larger, leaving the marks as a relative 'dot' in the bark. Simply put, the sculpting that when used up a huge share of the tree is now simply a small mark on a substantial tree-- simply a really little component of that tree's history.

Your errors are comparable. They may not disappear, however, as you get additional experiences, you are going to discover that you are able to bury them. They're a part of who you are, and in fact, you should not desire that differently-- nevertheless, they are a progressively unimportant part of who you are. The secret is to embrace them and grow anyhow.

Chapter 7: Compassion and Gratitude

There is a particular kind of remorse that is especially tough to let go, the kind where you blame yourself.

Therefore, another effective pointer for being calmer, happier and more satisfied? Sometimes simply cut yourself some slack. The majority of us are exceptionally rough on ourselves: more so than we ever would be with anybody else. We anticipate an excessive amount, and we do not permit basic slips or errors. Simply put: we require excellence and we seldom offer ourselves a break.

When was the final time you haven't completed as much work as you wished to? And how did you spend the remainder of that day? Probably, you regretted your imperfections and felt worried. Maybe you allow it to gnaw at your self-confidence, or you feel you aren't worthy of great things.

Now ask this: how would you have responded had somebody else informed you of those identical things? You'd, no question, have actually offered them a break and sympathized with them. So how about doing the identical thing with yourself?

This is an additional instance of mindfulness-- of being mindful of the examples of your thinking, and how those things impact your mood and mind. Is your thinking good? Or is it, in fact, rather harmful?

One method to alter your thoughts from a CBT viewpoint, is to attempt utilizing mantras. Mix this with post-it-notes around your house, which contain those notes so as to enhance your state of mind and prompt yourself to think more favorably. For this to function properly, those notes ought to be things that you currently think are correct to some level. So if you feel that you are smart, then compose a note telling yourself that.

Another extremely essential tip that you need to write in uppercase letters and put it where you are going to see it the initial moment you get up.

Kindness Toward Self

Journaling can assist too. Make a note of 3 things you did good today, and any compliments that individuals offered you. You can then check these out every now and then! This has a big effect, as for the majority of us, an insult has a much larger influence on our self-image than praise. This practice pushes you to alter that balance.

Kindness Meditation and Being Grateful

You may likewise practice being kinder to yourself with a thing referred to as 'caring kindness meditation.' This is a type of meditation that includes cultivating a sensation of compassion towards yourself. Indulge in that sensation, and let it truly sink in. Concentrate on this feeling and attempt to keep it for 10 minutes at once, a couple of times a week. It's genuinely transformative in the manner in which you see the world.

Lastly, think about cultivating a thankful mindset. This indicates concentrating on the important things you have, and the important things you are pleased with. This makes you more upbeat, and it brings you into the current moment and assists you to feel greater about the things that you have actually achieved. It's the best method to fight those sensations of remorse!

Within the journal, you ought to likewise make a note of 3 things that you are thankful for by the end of each day. This is going to push you to review just how much has actually gone well and just how much is great in your life.

Chapter 8: Bid Farewell to Social Stress And Anxiety

Social anxiety hamstring the lives of many individuals and can make it difficult for them to talk in public or perhaps engage with others in big social settings. While some individuals experience this sort of destructive impact, a lot more discover they have social anxiety to a lower extent, which may make them feel insecure in the work environment or amongst buddies. It can then stop them from meeting their potential in their professions or in their private lives.

Typically social anxiety boils down to a sensation that a person is, in some way insufficient, or that what they state isn't worth as much as what others have to say. Individuals decide not to talk since they fret that what they state is going to be 'dumb.' Simultaneously they fret that they may stumble or stutter, therefore, not getting their point across correctly.

One fast and simple method to enhance the clearness of your speech, in addition to your vocabulary, is to talk more gradually. The slower you speak, the more time you are going to have to consider the following thing you will say. It is going to likewise assist you in projecting your voice additionally, and you'll immediately sound deeper, clearer and more positive.

Use CBT to Be More Social

Nevertheless, if you remain in your own head, stressing over stuttering, then you'll discover this tough to do as you naturally talk faster when you're anxious. Paradoxically, it's fretting about getting a stutter that is going to give you a stutter. So how do you leave your own head sufficiently to talk more assuredly?

As we talked about at the beginning of this guide, in cognitive behavioral therapy, clients are informed to utilize what is called 'hypothesis testing.' Here you check the outcomes of doing anything it is you're nervous about in the hope that you discover that your worries are misguided. Remarkably, however, it might, in fact, be better if you discover that when you do say something dumb or stutter insanely, that there's absolutely nothing to be stressed over.

One manner in which you may check this is with complete strangers. Strike up a discussion in a bar, store or a coffee shop, and do not stress whatsoever about what you state or how. As a matter of fact, attempt talking as oddly as feasible about as boring a subject as feasible. You'll never ever see them again, so it matters not and it's simply a test. What you'll discover, however, is that they treat you equally as anybody else. Nicely and without accentuating your faults. That's humanity.

You see, everybody is too occupied stressing over how others view them to be in a position to judge anybody else. They are concerned about how you'll respond to what they have to state. If you require any more evidence that you're just as

legitimate and important person as they are--
there it is.

Chapter 9: Power of Environment

The suggestions in this guide can mainly be divided into 2 classifications: the components that look at assisting you to alter your psychology-- to value things more, and to be more kind to yourself; and the components that inform you to physically care for yourself.

Taking care of your hair, skin, and your health is going to all assist you to feel better and happier. You'll appear much healthier, and you are going to have a radiance that just comes along with self-satisfaction and self-confidence.

However, what about the environment? This is what gets ignored so frequently, however, individuals such as Marie Kondo show how essential this is to your general satisfaction and joy. Actually, altering your environment can influence your psychology in various manners and you can take advantage of any of these to be healthier and happier. Here are several things to think about.

Wonder and Awe

Here's one fantastic instance of how altering your environment can result in a better you: wonder and awe.

Picture being a prehistoric man and getting to the top of a mountain. Envision seeing valleys extending for miles before you. This allure and scope would leave you with wonder and awe. What's really taking place is that you are being pushed to reassess your location in the world-- which in turn is leading to big quantities of actual rewiring in your brain. This procedure happens together with an outpouring of neurotransmitters and hormones, which result in the sensation of spiritual sustenance we are all acquainted with.

When was the final time you observed something genuinely impressive that altered your point of view? Whether it's using a telescope or opting for a hike, search for instances of wonder. It might make your issues appear extremely little, all of a sudden.

Going on a vacation or journey and altering your environment can likewise assist you in conquering bad habits-- as our environment consists of triggers that make behaviors difficult to give up.

Nature Can Heal

Another incredible manner in which the environment can alter your sensations is by hanging out in nature. This is where we developed, and lavish natural surroundings once indicated an abundance of resources and food.

Therefore, opting for a walk in nature can have a comparable impact on us now—leading to a lowered heart rate and feeling of calm. As a matter of fact, lots of fantastic thinkers declare that choosing "nature walks" was what enabled them to come up with their finest concepts. Why? Due to the fact that we are more innovative when we are unwinded!

Your Living Space

Lastly, do not undervalue the unfavorable effect that a messy house can have on your frame of mind. If you can arrange and clean the area around you, then you can set off substantial modifications in your state of mind, efficiency, and more.

Keeping things simply a bit more minimal is among the most effective methods to do this, which typically suggests lowering mess. This likewise implies getting rid of the things that you do not definitely enjoy-- that do not bring you the most happiness-- which suggests that what is left are going to be just the important things that give you really good feelings.

While you ought to reduce then, you ought to likewise enhance quality. We have actually currently talked about how buying a better bathroom can assist you in taking greater care of yourself. The identical holds true of your living room, where a luxurious sofa can make a world of distinction. And it holds true of your bed room, where a gorgeous image can make you feel terrific.

Cash does not guarantee joy, however, treating yourself to lasting things that make you feel fantastic is one method to raise your spirits daily!

Chapter 10: The Truth About Self Esteem

I know a great deal of individuals who have nearly non-existent self-confidence, which I discover both distressing and hard to comprehend. I have actually been sharing and practicing these self-care ideas for several years! Let me inform you, it's definitely much better than self-loathing. The thing is that these individuals have a lot going for them that, and it opposes all reasoning.

One of them is liked by all our female buddies, has actually got a remarkable job working with celebs and exudes charm. A great deal of individuals would switch their bodies and lives for his and yet he informs me constantly that he does not see himself as in any way successful and does not 'appreciate' himself.

I'm not amongst those individuals who would switch lives. That does not indicate I do not appreciate features in him, however, I understand that other individuals most likely appreciate features in me. I, like them, have actually been provided with all the tools I require to be able to end up being whatever I wish to be.

So instead of hoping I was more like somebody, my time would be better invested, in fact, working towards ending up being more like them in that aspect. I can select the ideal aspects of everyone I appreciate and imitate them, and when you have actually got good at those things, you'll value them even more.

How to Be More Fit

Wish to be more charming? Be around other individuals more and improve your conversational style and posture.

View these set-backs not as a thing to get distressed about, however, as obstacles. Envision you're in the Rocky movie -- a montage begins and you train up until you're fantastic at the important things you wish to be terrific at. I once wished to trade my life with stars who had discovered love and success – however, the adventure is all in the chase.

in case you work your way up to the top, you can delight in it correctly with the feeling of point of view that it needed to arrive. The moment you begin working towards an objective such as this you have a purpose and a goal, and you're not a 'no one' any longer.

So there genuinely is no requirement to be dissatisfied with yourself. If you're dissatisfied with an element of yourself, then alter it. The important thing is, nobody understands what the point of life is, so how can anybody inform you you're not doing it correctly? Somebody who's made no cash might think about themselves as a failure, however, if they have a great deal of family and friends, and have lead a complete life, then who can say they are failing? As long as you go after what you take pleasure in, that's what matters.

In addition, nobody ought to evaluate anybody else on their behavior due to the fact that they can't truly understand what's happening in that individual's life. If you're acting abnormally, maybe you're experiencing difficulty in your private life. The genuine point is not to defer to the acceptance of others and not to allow it to govern you. Just you can evaluate the worth of what you do. Stick to your own beliefs in your own manner, and you are going to achieve success in your own eyes.

Conclusion

I hope that, in the process, you have actually learned a little bit about the significance of self-love and self-care, and possibly what has actually caused tension and low self-confidence to begin with.

Today it's time to take the theory and transform it into something useful. From all we have actually found out, here is your plan to a better and more satisfied you:

- Utilize mindfulness to comprehend your self-talk more

- Put mantras around the house informing yourself of your finest qualities and to 'be nice' to oneself

- Take care of your look-- spend time, effort, and money on your appearance

- Attempt meditating

- Take care of your health by working out routinely in a manner that is maintainable and light

- Dress nicely

- Have a grooming routine and delight in the procedure as much as the result

- Obtain 8 hours of quality sleep each night

- Consume healthy food

- Hang around with individuals you like, practice the important things you aren't yet good at

- Clean your living space

- Go on vacations, look for instances of wonder and awe

- Surround yourself with stunning things that you like

- Maintain a journal and utilize it to jot down things that you are thankful for, and things you have actually done properly

Take all these actions daily, and you are going to be certain to delight in sensations of satisfaction and self-love.

I hope that you enjoyed reading through this book and that you have found it useful. If you want to share your thoughts on this book, you can do so by leaving a review on the Amazon page. Have a great rest of the day.

Printed in Great Britain
by Amazon